Why Are You Reading This?

You may think the idea of training with a bag of sand may be a bit crazy. You may be wondering why would I train with such a thing, could it be really that BIG of a difference? Heck, I have a whole gym full of equipment available to me, why in the world would I even CONSIDER sandbag training? Let's face it, if you are reading this right now you aren't happy with your results. You know they could be better, but you may not be sure what is missing from your programs.

I'll be honest, sandbags themselves will not solve your problems. I can tell you this from personal experience as I had high hopes for using sandbags for my own issues. My goal was to find training methods that could help my low back, which I had suffered a severe injury during my athletic career." Being so frustrated with the failure of traditional therapeutic techniques I had to search for something outside of the norm."

Immensely frustrated by the lack of progress in my own training and results I came across something very unusual. I began to study the work of old time strongman techniques. These great men believed in an idea of "Physical Culture". These athletes were not just performing feats of strength that would be impressive by today's standards. Yet, they were not just strong, but could move with the grace that would make the most elite athlete's jaw drop. What secrets did they know that we do not?

It was a challenge to identify what made them so successful as they all had their own unique methods and ideas, I couldn't find any specific commonalities except for one! At one point or another it appeared that most of these old time strongmen lifted odd objects. Stones, giant logs, and large bags of a variety of implements. This all seemed counterproductive to someone who had the history of low back pain that I had experienced, yet, I was desperate! I needed SOMETHING that would make a profound difference for pain and discomfort, I simply could not go on living life in this manner.

I didn't want to use everything, I was hesitant and thought of the odd objects discussed by old-time strongmen which made the most sense? Heck, I wasn't even sold that such a thing would make a difference for me. Exploring the idea of odd objects to a deeper level it appeared that even some of the strongmen had their favorites. In fact, one of the most popular modern proponents of Physical Culture, Brooke Kubik, spoke very specifically about the benefits of sandbag training and improving the body's strength and health.

"you feel sore because the bags (sandbags) worked your body in ways you could not approach with a barbell alone. You got into the muscle areas you normally don't work. You worked the "heck" out of the stabilizers." (Kubik, p. 115)

STABILIZERS, this was something with background in Exercise Science and Corrective Exercise I understood and greatly appreciated. I knew that a lot of my own problems had to do with weakness in stabilizers and although I had placed great emphasis in building up the supporting structures of my body, I wasn't sure if I was hitting on the most meaningful stabilizers that would actually impact my low back.

Even with hesitation I knew my current training wasn't doing the job and I had only one choice. I threw myself in the fire and built my first sandbag. Yes, out of the old duffel bag and garbage bags. I remember once duct taping the top I was ready to give it a whirl and see if sandbag training was something that had legs. Even from rep one of the first lift I was sold. This was unlike ANYTHING I had lifted in the past. Especially not being a novice to a lot of forms of strength training, this was different. I felt weak, I felt muscles trying to work that I had never felt, and comparable to the barbell this was a "light" weight.

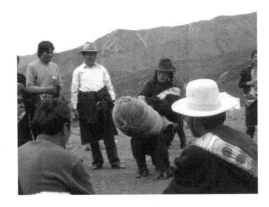

Yes, I was sold within minutes. I started trying to lift my homemade sandbag every way possible. Every repetition felt like a new exercise and I began to feel my core fire in ways that were completely new to me. After even a few sessions of working the sandbags into my routines I felt myself standing taller, my postural muscles seemed to be renewed, and most of all I was beginning to see the some significant differences in my low back pain and stability.

This was exciting, immediately I knew that this was something I wanted my clients to experience as well. One of the biggest weaknesses for anyone is the stabilizers and usually those are muscles in the hips, abdominals, low back, and shoulders. Interestingly many of the same areas that most people get injured. My sandbag program was ready to roll and be implemented in all of my clients' workouts. I had created a host of different weights to accommodate all my clients. This was going to be exciting, dynamic, and best of all have people experience the same changes I had felt myself.

The Failure of a Great Idea!

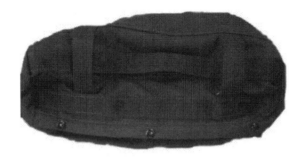

My hopes in using the homemade sandbags with my clients quickly went downhill. My clients found the homemade sandbags to be clumsy, they didn't allow them to learn how to progressively move better. It became messy and ultimately non-productive to their goals. In actually trying to implement the sandbags with my clients I learned that it felt like we were trying to replicate barbell work, and it appeared sloppy. It was not providing them the success I anticipated. Ironically, I found myself hitting a plateau with the sandbag training. My enthusiasm began to fall and I thought shortly I would have to move on to other training ideas. Maybe I had maximized the full potential of the sandbag. As others have found it was a great complimentary tool, but sandbag would never be the focus and foundation of my fitness programs.

I began using the sandbags less and less, ripped knuckles, dirty training areas, and lack of progression began to sour me on sandbags. Maybe they were just the occasional "shock your body" type of training. However, it dawned on me that we were hoping that magically a training implement would solve all our fitness needs. What a flaw in thinking as a fitness coach, I was ashamed that I fell into the simple trap of such an obvious problem. Just because you give someone a paint brush doesn't mean they create beautiful paintings. The question became, "was it the sandbag or the way we thought of the sandbag that halted results?"

A Revelation and a New Journey

The base concept that the sandbag could hit the body in ways nothing else could made me think there had to be a manner to implement a better training tool. Right off I knew we could NOT be using homemade equipment. Heck, the more I thought about it the more outrageous using homemade equipment actually seemed. I never looked around the gym and found objects that people created. There weren't homemade barbells, dumbbells, kettlebells, bands, or even medicine balls. I would never use a homemade piece of equipment for anything in life that I demanded a great outcome from. My mind got busy on how could I make sandbag training more accessible to more people and instead of a training implement, make it a system of fitness and performance training.

The first step was making a sandbag to meet the demands of our training. I knew absolutely NOTHING about manufacturing, I did know what I wanted. A new training system had to address the following needs:

- Progressive

- Versatile

- Based Upon Solving Problems

- That meant I had solved the many problems that traditional sandbags had possessed.

- Couldn't Control The Dimensions of the Bag

- Didn't Have Multiple Options in Developing Progressive Exercises

- Weren't Designed to Move in Many Patterns and Positions

The VERY first Ultimate Sandbags™ developed in 2005 solved many of these problems. There were three sizes that allowed us to not only control the weight but the dimension of the Ultimate Sandbag™. This was important as there would be times we wanted to have a sandbag that moved less and times we wanted the weight to shift more. There would be moments in training where using a smaller, more compact Ultimate Sandbag™ was ideal. Other times a larger dimension Ultimate Sandbag™ would solve the problem.

Training vs. Exercises Just Semantics?

Having a specifically designed Ultimate Sandbag™ is only part of the equation. Even the best tools don't produce much if they are not used correctly and effectively. Can you screw up using Ultimate Sandbags™ though? Aren't they just "bags of sand?" Don't worry, even the pros mistake the idea that Ultimate Sandbag™ Training is impossible to perform incorrectly. In a Men's Fitness article it was written;

"Don't be overly concerned about form-the sand will shift around, making it hard to control the bag. That's the point. Having to stabilize yourself constantly will work you from head to toe."

Such thinking as described in the quote above demonstrates the problem if we don't truly understand what we are trying to accomplish through this very unique form of training. In fact, if an implement like an Ultimate Sandbag™ moves and shifts during a lift then it is even more important that the lifter both understand and perform proper technique because every repetition is going to be distinctly different.

Part of the problem is that people can't quite wrap their head around the idea of a "bag of sand" creating superior fitness. This is actually quite odd when you consider the fact that most of the best fitness tools are not more complex in their design and often quite the opposite. If we were to examine barbells, they are simply long pieces of metal we place circular pieces of metal upon. Dumbbells have even less design as they are only a portion of barbells. Medicine balls are overgrown bouncy balls, stability balls are stronger inflatable beach balls. Even kettlebells that have become mainstream in today's fitness culture are even described by those that endorse them as "cannon balls with handles." It may be surprising to think that the Ultimate Sandbag is designed to meet specific needs of fitness programs which is greatly different than most training tools. Unfortunately, we far too often conform our training to the training tool and not use the training tool as the solution to our fitness goals. We should make the tool work for us, not the other way around!

Once we see our fitness tools in these terms it may actually seem very reasonable and even exciting to have a dynamic implement specifically designed for the goals of fitness and performance based training. However, even if you are ready to go train with Ultimate Sandbags™ right away I just can't let you! You see most people do get this positive excitement and then it hits them, "what am I suppose to do with Ultimate Sandbags™ anyway?"

Sure, you could hit some barbell type lifts for a little bit, but as I experienced without a purpose your training will inevitably plateau. That is why you have to understand the system, the purpose behind the training. Let's get away from the idea of sandbags and even the Ultimate Sandbag™ and think how Dynamic Variable Resistance Training™ (DVRT) will deliver what I promise.

Knowledge Really Is Power

Fortune 500 corporations, elite military programs, complex architecture design, what do they have in common? They are only as successful as the plans they create, a system of creating their success. A successful business is never randomly built, an extensive business plan is created to give direction, focus, and problem solving. Same with the military, soldiers aren't randomly thrown into battle with no plan. Buildings are never randomly put together in hopes that it will hold together. If these situations all have models and plans then why don't we do the same for the complex system that is our body.

Some people are fearful that plans and programs are stale and stagnant. That programs and systems will take all the "fun" out of training, can't we just make it play? As Strength Coach, Charles Staley, says, "you can't deviate from a system you don't have!" A training program and system is simply a plan. It gives you direction, focus, and the ability to problem solve when things aren't going right. Far too many people are just doing "stuff" and while doing different things all the time satisfies our exercise A.D.D., such training usually doesn't allow us to achieve our fitness goals.

What makes the Dynamic Variable Resistance Training™ (DVRT™) a worthwhile system, different from other fitness programs? As Speed Expert, Lee Taft, states effective training is about teaching "skills not drills." Most fitness programs are based around exercises even if they claim not to be. The skill of teaching movement is often talked about but rarely taught in a progressive manner.

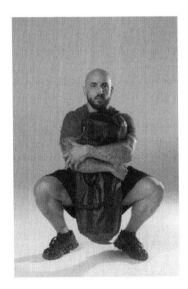

Let's take the movement of squatting. A movement pattern we know is very important in developing both strength and mobility. Yet, speak to most people in the gym about squatting and you will get moans and groans from the achy backs and knees that many experience with squatting under the bar. In the fitness industry we realize the need to teach people to perform the squat well, yet, we generally have two schools of thought on this foundational movement pattern. One will breakdown the squat into many individual "corrective" exercises that are supposedly going to help you squat better. Don't worry, it may only take you 8 to 12 weeks till you see the "possible" impact of these drills. Or, you may find those that feel if you just "keeping doing it" somehow you will get better. Either mentality doesn't seem to be the most effective nor efficient.

The DVRT™ System provides strategies to solve many of these problems. With our squatting progressions set forth in the DVRT™ Program, we can use our foundational exercises to immediately improve squatting performance and at the same time increase strength in the movement that we are trying to develop. Our drills in the DVRT™ system crossover many areas of fitness often providing many qualities to be developed at once. It is not unusual for a DVRT™ series of progressions to develop strength, stability, endurance, core strength, be corrective, and be highly effective for fat loss. Sounds too good to be true, but we will delve deeper into the program and give you workouts to experience for yourself the power of this unique training system and how it applies to a great variety of movement patterns that can enhance your fitness, strength and health!

Our DVRT™ transforms how we see foundational movement patterns as well. While some programs may be excited that they have 3 or 4 different ways to squat, the DVRT™ program can have up to 12 different squatting variations. This allows great progression and no excuse for ever becoming "bored" with your fitness program.

Squatting

The ability to squat well is actually NOT a prerequisite of training in the DVRT™ system. In fact, the Ultimate Sandbag™ (USB™) can serve as a means of improving quality of movement in foundational drills such as squatting. Being able to squat well should be a goal of every coach and lifter, however, what makes a "good" squat is going to be based on several factors.

- Neural Control

- Joint Movement

- Soft-tissue Restrictions

The last two can often be a challenge to change immediately, however, changing neural control during a lift is one of the easiest and most powerful components to change. We see such changes all the time during training programs in the form of rapid increases in strength of practiced lifts. Because muscular changes often take 6-8 weeks we know that these fast improvements are largely due to neurological changes in coordination of muscle fibers, motor units, and the body's ability to coordinate the muscles to perform a movement more efficiently.

In order to allow a lifter to learn correct postures, loading through the body, and remove negative leverage to their body we can begin to improve their squatting ability by going through our positional loading progressions.

Bear Hug Squat:

The position of the USB™ in the Bear Hug Squat keeps the body's center of gravity at a standard level. This means that the body's balance will not be thrown off by the additional load added to it. In fact, the Bear Hug position will act as a counter balance to the lifter's body allowing a more upright posture to be maintained during all squatting motions. The upright posture is important as it will both reduce load on the low back and make the lifter stay on their heels, both key concepts in performing proper squats.

The additional benefit of using the USB™ Bear Hug Squat is the isometric upper body strength. The extensors of the thoracic spine will be challenged demonstrating any type of weakness in the postural muscles as well as poor motor patterns. Far too many people have their upper back round which also means the low back gets into a compromised position causing excessive loading on the lumbar spine. We can correct this by using the Bear Hug Squat to reinforce these muscles to be active and will help maintain alignment of not just the upper back, but the lower back as well. This means ANYONE not only can learn how to squat correctly but we can help chronic postural problems as well.

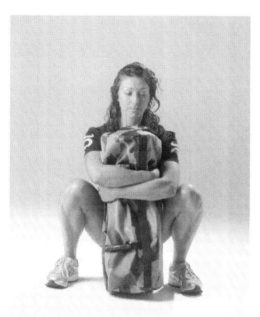 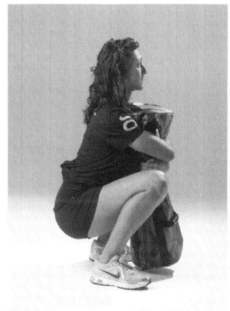

Zercher Squat:

The Zercher squat is used as a means to change the perceived weight of the USB™. Making what outwardly seems to be a modest change in the holding position of the USB™ greatly changes the perceived weight as the center of gravity is raised on the body as well as increase stress to the core and upper back muscles.

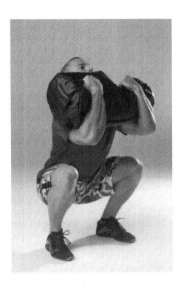

A large benefit of the Zercher squat is the amount of core training that this position and exercise provides. The Zercher position often is missed as being very similar to the core stabilization exercise of being in a plank position on the ground. Performing Zercher lifts offers some advantages that floor planks do not.

• For advanced trainees it is important to learn how to maintain posture during dynamic motion especially as your base of support diminishes.

• Sometimes both elderly and beginners can find getting up and down from the ground can be excessive. Introducing this type of training for those populations can provide the desired core training while still supporting a positive training experience.

The key in the Zercher Squat is to make sure the upper back doesn't round which will definitely lead to low back rounding. Great core strength is represented by the ability to keep the chest tall and no rounding. It is obvious we can make the core work hard in the Zercher Squat by going heavier, but that is far from the only way! Another terrific way to really challenge the core during the Zercher squat is to slow the repetitions down...way down! The slower you can take the lowering aspect of the Zercher Squat the more you will find the core working hard to keep your posture and alignment. This demonstrates great core strength and control which should be a precursor to adding any additional weight to the exercise.

The Staggered Squat

It might surprise people not see the standard squatting and then lunging progression. In our DVRT system we teach an intermediate step that really helps people achieve far greater results. The Staggered Squat is a solution to a lot of people's needs of balancing adding more weight, but also improving stability.

What is the Staggered Squat? If we take our squat stance and slowly move one foot back so the back toes are in line with the front foot's heel, that is the basis of our Staggered Squat. The difference is not just in the foot alignment, but the fact the back foot has only the ball of foot in contact with the ground. The means we are putting more work into the front leg and combining a more progressive means in teaching single leg training. Just as we wouldn't add massive weight from set to set, taking someone from a squat to lunge position is the equivalent of doing just so!

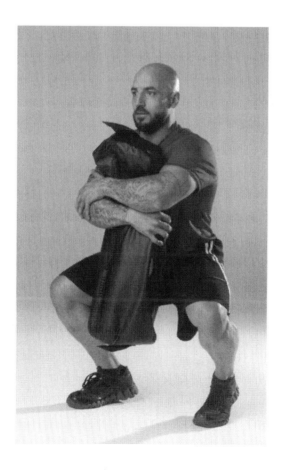

The Staggered Squat allows people to learn how to properly stabilize on one leg without being overwhelmed, or worse being exposed to exercises that are too advanced. A often overlooked benefit to the Staggered Squat is that it can be a starting place for people that suffer flexibility issues. By opening the hips, people can begin to start learning the squat position while at the same time working on improving the mobility in their lower body. Another opportunity to build success in the DVRT system.

Shoulder Squat:

The Shoulder Squat is the most popular of USB™ lifts, but is often done incorrectly and without proper purpose. This squatting variation places the greatest demand on the lateral stability of the body. It takes what is largely a sagittal plane movement and places severe demands in both the frontal and transverse planes. This gives even MORE value to the squatting motion as our squat becomes a true 3-dimensional squat vs 3 dimensional.

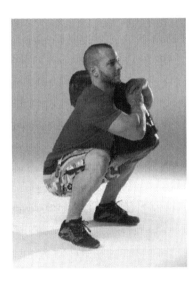

As we can make a parallel of the Zercher squat to the plank exercise, we can likewise make a similar parallel of the Shoulder Squat to the side plank. The Shoulder Squat not only is a performance based movement, but allows us to assess an individual in a relatively safe and easy to learn format. Lack of stability through the trunk and pelvis will present itself in movement of the pelvis to one side versus another during the lower or ascending phase of the squat. This will provide important feedback to the coach to the level of true "core stabilization."

Additionally, because one side of the body is working significantly harder than the opposing, the Shoulder Squat serves as a great progression to beginning lifters that are trying trying to progress towards unilateral lower body training and more advanced core stabilization.

Note: Although there are 12 squatting variations in the DVRT™ System we are discussing the most important and foundational 7 DVRT™ Squatting Movements: Bear Hug->Zercher->Shoulder->Bear Hug Staggered->Zercher Staggered->Rear Shoulder Staggered->Same Shoulder Staggered. Please visit www.DVRTFtiness.com for more resources on all our squatting variations, or take one of our world renown educational courses with newly updated programs all the time at www.DVRTFitness.com.

Explosive Training

A great benefit to the DVRT™ system is the fact that every lift must begin with getting the weight off the ground. Depending upon the receiving position of the USB™, we will have to alter our position and challenge our mobility in different ways . Always make sure that proper lifting technique is instilled before ever approaching more advanced deliberate rounded back lifting.

Lifting the USB™ from the ground gives a great opportunity to teach people the difference between hip hinging and squatting. This is an essential component to proper lifting and low back safety. Many people are still told to save their low backs by squatting to pick-up objects from the ground. This is actually incorrect as your glutes and hamstrings are far stronger than your quadriceps and are meant for producing a great amount of force. "Hinging" at the hips is a necessary technique not to just perform exercises but teaches people correct movement skills that will be applied in everyday life. There is another important reason that explosive exercises are performed in the DVRT™ System. Explosive USB™ exercises can be a form of high intensity interval training for many people that have found other forms of training to be troublesome on their knees and low back such as running. Short bursts of intense activity like those that are used in the DVRT™ programs have been shown to be a SUPERIOR way to lose fat to traditional "cardio" training. However, because many activities such as running and jumping can cause people discomfort they never embrace high intensity interval training (HIIT).

Using the following USB™ exercises is a terrific means to not only accomplish the fat loss training effect of HIIT training, but because there is a great emphasis on strengthening the hamstrings, hips, and core we can concurrently be improving achy knees and troublesome low backs. (NOTE: Make sure to check with your physician before performing any fitness program and those outlined in this book).

How to Accelerate Well!

Bringing the USB™ to a lifting position becomes an explosive drill because the weight must be accelerated to the proper holding position. The USB™ accelerative/explosive drills are closely related to the barbell in many ways and provide some unique attributes as well. Many of the benefits of Olympic weightlifting come in the form of what is know as triple extension. This natural movement pattern of the body means that the ankle/foot, knee, and hip quickly extend to develop force upwards to the body. Think of trying to jump as high as you can and you will see how your body naturally produces this movement. Triple extension refers to the ankle, knee, and hip all extending in one synergistic movement. This helps the body to develop power, but why develop power if you aren't an athlete? Learning how to utilize this triple extension and power of the body helps take load off the low back. So next time you are loading something heavy into your car, moving furniture on the weekend, you will appreciate learning this powerful movement."

Yet, Olympic lifting can often be challenging to coach and learn. Factor in as well Olympic lifting is a sport based around certain drills and not meant for the progressive fitness training that many people require to be both successful and safe. What is "early pulling of the arms?" Many times when people are learning a new movement or feeling challenged in the weight they are using, they find ways to cheat! In most situations the body will try to leverage what it perceives to be the strongest parts of the body, in this case the upper body. The truth is that the lower body is far stronger and if you follow the correct technique you will both be able to lift more weight and do it more safely. Pulling the arms early means that one begins to bend the elbows before the weight starts to move. The elbows should only move when the USB is being accelerated.

Bear Hug:

The explosive Bear Hug pull is an essential placement exercise and because of the end point being the lowest to the body to the other explosive variations. Because the weight travels a shorter distance this means that we have to produce the least amount of force to get the USB™ in the correct position. A great teaching tool for those that are learning how to accelerate a weight off the ground.

Placement of the USB™ is paramount as the lifter should stand 50% over the USB, moving too far behind the USB™ can cause the lifter to overload the low back. The lifter either staggers the hands or interlocks the fingers, on smaller USB™s interlocking the hands is ideal while on large USB™s using the staggered hand position creates more surface area and control for the lifter.

With the hips hinging back lower the body into proper lifting posture without rounding the low back. The explosive makes the USB™ weightless and pulls directly into the Bear Hug holding position. Using excessive power will make the USB™ hit the body excessively instead of "floating" into the correct holding position.

Power Clean:

The Power Clean takes the USB™ from the vertical to horizontal position in front of the body. This position appears much closer to the more familiar barbell Power Clean. However, the grip is a parallel grip instead of the pronated version found on the barbell. By taking the parallel handle position it is easier to lock in the upper body and create a more stable foundation for driving with the hips. The Power Clean with the USB™ requires us to produce more force and therefore gets the user to perform the triple extension which is essential to avoid excessive lower back loading.

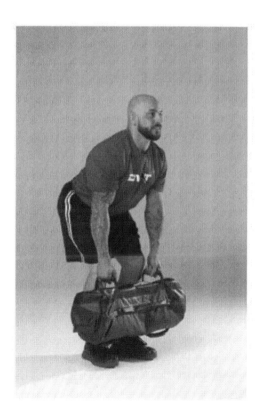 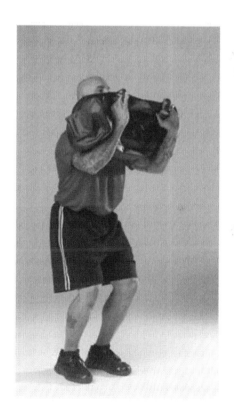

The USB™ must start as close to the shins as possible, this reduces stress upon the low back. Because the weight of the USB™ will begin to drop away from the lifters as they begin to pull the weight off the floor it is important to watch for early pulling of the arms.

The movement should involve no arm tension while the lifter creates enough force that the arms can "sweep" under the weight to catch the USB™ in the crooks of the arms. Failure to create enough force the lifter will find the weight to stall and won't be able to get the arms around the USB™. Full extension of the body should occur from deliberately driving high forces into the ground.

To reverse the movement the lifter must unwind the body by beginning with a slight chest bump to get the USB™ moving off the body. The "bump" must not drive the USB™ too far away from the body, it is just enough to begin the movement of unwinding the body, if the elbows come away from the rib cage the push was too hard. A good rule is to always have the elbows close to the body both on the acceleration and deceleration of the weight.

The lifter must absorb the downward momentum by keeping the USB™ close to the body and quickly dropping the hips back into the original lifting position. Not cueing this rapid downward pull of the body makes the dropping force of the USB™ very large on the shoulders and lower back.

Shouldering:

Of all the movements that are familiar to sandbag training, none may be more powerful than Shouldering. Having said that, there are few drills that are improperly performed than Shouldering exercises. Most of this is due to the fact that lifters and coaches focus only on the fact of getting the USB™ to the shoulder and NOT how it is done. As mentioned in previous sections, as the instability of lifting rises, technical components of the lift become even more critical.

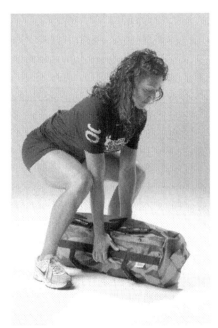
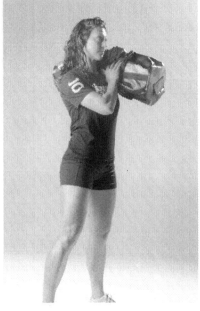

Shouldering does represent the most unstable of all the USB™ base power movements. This is due to two factors:

- As the lifter begins the movement and accelerate the USB™ off the ground, the load will actually move away from the lifter making them rely even more on proper hip drive. It will be very important to have proper sequence of hip movement to avoid having all the load being driven into the low back and upper body.

- The placement of the load is usually overlooked. In previous discussions of Shouldering movements, this challenges the frontal and transverse planes of stability greatly. An inability to stabilize in these planes can show themselves in great compensations especially in the pelvis. Additionally, Shouldering requires the most power as half the USB™ must clear the shoulder. This is higher than even the barbell in the standard clean. Many lifters make the mistake of not performing the full lift.

As with most lifts, Shouldering is largely based upon taking the correct lifting position before the load is ever attempted to be moved. Straddling the USB™ so that half is behind and half is in front is the ideal position allowing equal distribution of weight. Far too often lifters will allow too much of the USB™ to be out in front of them resulting in excessive load in the low back. Such mistakes commonly occur during repetition work as the USB™ will start to "creep" out in front of the lifter as they drop it back down to the ground. Repositioning is paramount for safety and proper training.

Lifting the USB™ in Shouldering can occur from the ground or knee height. More load can be lifted from the ground and this is typically an easier learning position for most lifters. Lifting from the knee is great for developing more explosive power or repetition work because the range of motion is decreased. Similar to the Bear Hug lift, determining proper starting height is important in preventing injury and ensuring proper lifting postures. Because the load will start so low to the ground the lifter and/or coach needs to ensure that squatting or rounding of the back does not occur in initial stages of training. Rounded back lifting is a form of advanced USB™ training and not recommended for the majority of fitness enthusiasts..

In all explosive USB™ lifting the arms need to be thought of as simply an extension of the hips. Because the USB™ will begin to drop against the lifter during Shouldering there is a natural tendency to pull with the arms either at the beginning of the movement or when many lifters "stall" at approximately hip height because they didn't generate enough force with the hips. Extension of the entire body must occur to elevate the USB™ to the point of comfortably clearing the shoulder.

Absorbing the force and returning the USB™ to the start position are two critical components as well. To properly absorb the load of the USB™ the lifter should "catch" the USB™ with a quarter squat. This technique removes some of the impact of the USB™ to the body and makes it a more comfortable lift. Catching the USB™ with locked legs is acceptable, but may cause more impact for the lifter. Returning the USB™ to the start is similar to the other explosive lifts. A "bump" off the shoulder will initiate the movement, however, the lifter will have to direct the weight making sure the load stays close to the body. Having the arms extending away from the rib cage indicates that the load is getting away from the lifter and may have excessive force upon the low back.

The low back is not the only point of consideration during the eccentric phase of Shouldering. Many lifters and coaches forget the impact of the upper body as well. Catching the USB™ during the eccentric phase can cause high loads in the shoulders and arms. It is necessary for the lifter to maintain tension in the upper back to create a stable foundation for the upper body to absorb the force of the USB™ coming downwards. Being "loose" in the upper body can create a "yanking" action that can lead to problems in the shoulders and elbows.

The Foundation of DVRT™ Upper Body Training: Overhead Pressing

Before the time of bench presses and racks, strength was measured by how much weight someone could put overhead. In many ways this old time measure was probably a better predictor of true whole body strength than the more muscles of the body have to work together to perform the movement well. While the body is supported in cases like the bench press it is easy to have key muscles of the body relax because the body is receiving an external support.

Not having an external support means that the whole body must contribute to the goal of lifting overhead. Think of a building with a weak foundation, it won't be able to remain strong and last for a long time. The same thing is with the body, a weak foundation from the lower body or core will make the upper body feel weak and compromise the quality of an overhead exercise. That is why it is important to distinguish the fact that these are NOT "shoulder" drills rather overhead exercises because the shoulders are only a very small part of the equation.

Unique Aspects of DVRT™ Overhead Pressing

The USB™ offers two different strategies to pressing overhead. The first being the more stable is the bilateral neutral grip press. The press is completely predicated upon the clean of the USB™.

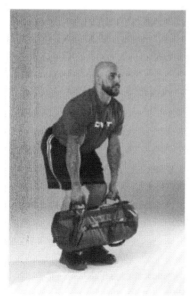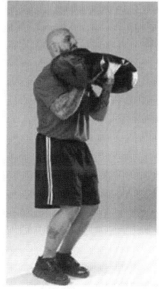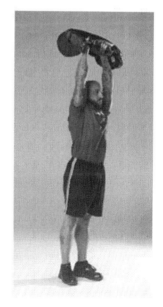

An improper clean will lead to the lifter expending excessive time recovering the load and creating too much fatigue to maximize pressing power. Therefore, consideration must given on the type of USB ™ used.

To perform overhead pressing the USB™ must land on top of the fists in a neutral position. The USB™ should NOT be on the back side or front side of the wrists during any portion of the press. Such a technique will lead to excessive strain on the shoulders as well as the wrists. Because the USB™ moves and shifts many lifters mistakenly allow the USB™ to shift to these improper loading positions. Because of the resting position of the weight, a larger USB™ that is more loosely loaded is better than a very tight USB™ because the shape of the USB™ changes to more of a rounded shape making proper cleaning very difficult. This is a situation where understanding the training tool becomes very important in proper performing the movement properly. More tightly filled USB™s will be used during the other pressing variation.

The clean and press of the USB™ carries many similar principles as those of the kettlebell. A good clean will result in the lifter creating a stable base by actively locking the legs by driving the feet into the ground. By then creating compression through the torso the lifter drives the weight overhead by pushing with the lats. Keeping in the arms in the neutral position allows those lifters that traditionally have shoulder problems have less pain. Additionally, the neutral position makes it easier for the coach to teach the press from the lats and trunk rather than the upper traps or just deltoids.

Pressing the USB™ from this position allows us to apply the most amount of weight, or to introduce overhead lifting to people starting a fitness program as it is a more balanced lifting position. With the weight off the USB™ on the fists we also find some unique attributes of DVRT™. The weight will often feel uneven between the hands making it increasingly more demanding upon our core to hold good postural alignment as we lift the USB™ overhead. This same instability also means that the shoulder stabilizers are working hard and while we are getting stronger we are also helping prevent future injury of the shoulder joint.

NOTE: The Power USB is actually pressed from the outside handles to place the body in a better alignment for the shoulders.

Shoulder to Shoulder Press

Outwardly it would appear that single arm pressing is not an option on the USB™ (pressing from the single handle is not often recommended), yet, we can reposition the USB™ to create some very unique and powerful single arm pressing variations. By changing the alignment of the

USB™ on the shoulder where even though two arms are on the USB™ only one has the leverage to actually create a pressing motion.

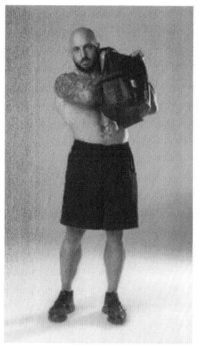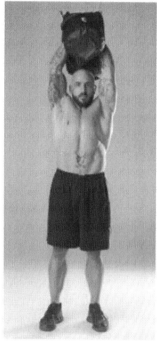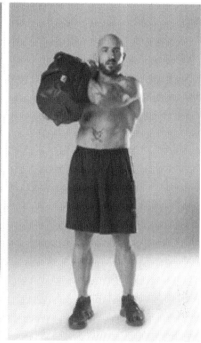

This creates a unique single arm pressing drill because it will provide instant feedback upon movement compensations and transition of the body's center of gravity. The compensations occur if the lifter does not properly load the lat that is on the side of the USB™. Not performing this results in the elbow of the pressing arm to "wing" and/or the upper trap to shrug the shoulder upwards, both demonstrate a lack of control of the pressing movement.

These compensations not only key into the fact the lifter is not properly loading the lat, but there are issues in the chain of the entire frontal plane stabilizers. These stabilizers are critical in increasing performance and decreasing risk of injury. Such imbalances would appear in leveraging the hip or moving the body away from either side of the press. Symmetry should be strived for in the Shoulder to Shoulder Press.

As the lifter presses from shoulder to shoulder the center of gravity through the body changes increasing the body's need to change it patterns of stability throughout the movement creating a more functional form of core training. The key is to strive for the same quality of press that would be performed with other training implements. This is referring to complete press out of the arms overhead and not changing posture at any level of the movement.

Ultimate Sandbag™ Progressions

All of the fundamental movement patterns of USB™ training can be progressed by changing a series of different variables. Most coaches and lifters simply focus upon changing the load of the specific lift. While this is a viable option, in may prove less than optimal for those that are training in group or team situations. It also becomes limiting with the USB™ to only focus on load. Similar to implements such as kettlebells, the USB can jump too fast in weight increments, making progression seem outwardly challenging. However, like kettlebells, altering other variables such as leverage and load position not only solve such problems but give the USB an advantage over other training implements.

Therefore, we have several other options (along with load) to create positive training progressions and programs. As discussed in the early section of this manual, changing the holding position of the USB™ is one of the easiest means of adjusting perceived load to the lifter. Refer to the early chapter to work through proper holding positions with the USB™.

A preferred method for adjusting overload is to also change the body position of the lifter. This principle can be applied very similarly for upper body and lower body emphasized lifts. These variations for the different foundational lifts are reviewed below.

Squatting

• Bear Hug Bilateral	• Zercher Staggered Stance
• Zercher Bilateral	• Clean Staggered Stance
• Clean Bilateral	• USB on Back Foot Shoulder Staggered Stance
• Shoulder Bilateral	• USB on Side of Stance Leg Staggered Stance
• Bear Hug Staggered Stance	

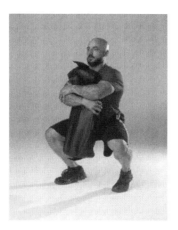

While such a list of progressions may at first appear overwhelming, the truth is they allow us a better opportunity to succeed with our training. We can improve our strength and fitness by not just lifting bigger weights, but improving our stability and mobility as well. Therefore, we can find the "RIGHT" progression and exercise for your fitness goal and level." This allows us to not only customize your current fitness program, but progress to so many variations boredom is never an option!

The DVRT philosophy moves from stable to unstable. One of the easiest ways to see this progression is moving from squatting to single leg exercises. The lunge is such a classic, but misunderstood exercise and like many other movements, DVRT will re-invent it for your training!

Lunging has many progressions beyond just using one's body weight or tiny dumbbells. One way is the direction that people lunge:

• Static Lunge

• Reverse Lunge

• Forward Lunge

• Lateral Static Lunge

• Crossover Lunge

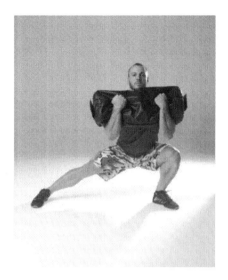

One can go through the same progression holding as in the squatting patterns, but being on the single leg actually provides us with many useable options such as the following USB™ holding positions including; down by the hip, headlock, behind the neck, and overhead positions.

The point to be taken is the amount of variations and options a coach and/or lifter has in designing programs and addressing specific needs even if they exist in a class or team format. Unfortunately, most of these types of progressions are only in terms of the lower body, meanwhile, the upper body drills could benefit from viewing progressions in a similar manner. This would actually accelerate success in strength and stability gains.

We have a host of options as well for the upper body by manipulating both the position of the USB™ and our body position. As with all our progressions we want to change only one variable at a time otherwise the intensity of the exercise can become too high.

Bilateral Neutral Grip/ Shoulder to Shoulder Press Progressions

- Bilateral Stance
- Staggered Stance
- Rear Foot Elevated
- Top of Lunge
- Half Kneeling
- Bottom of Lunge
- Suspended

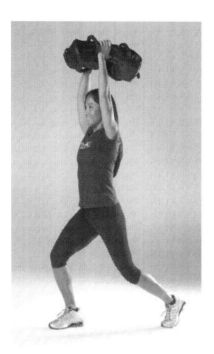

While the progressions are the same for both the neutral grip press and the shoulder to shoulder press, it is significantly more challenging to perform these movements with the shoulder to shoulder press because of the changing frontal plane stability demands as the USB™ is moving overhead side to side in unstable positions. Additionally we have to remember that even though two hands are on the USB™ during the shoulder to shoulder press only one arm is really lifting the weight.

This goes without looking into factors such as changing speed or range of motion as well. Opening up these other factors simply expands the options and means to increase strength for the lifter especially as they begin to be combined. Creating more options can sometimes appear overwhelming, but as they are put into practice the experience of using these techniques helps accelerate progress not just in performance, but in resiliency against injury.

Advanced DVRT™ Exercises-Rotational Skills

The most exciting aspect of Ultimate Sandbag™ training is the fact we have so many more options to create dynamic exercise programs due to the flexibility of the Ultimate Sandbag™. A perfect example of creating more sophisticated training is the progression to adding complexity to Ultimate Sandbag™ movements.

We can accomplish this goal by continuing to alter body position in the form of adding rotation. Our muscles and bodies are meant to rotate especially if we think about very functional movements such as throwing, kicking, punching, and how we can create the most amount of force. However, adding complexity also means also means we need to be in more control of our movement patterns. The foundational exercises provide us the ability to learn how to perform these more complex patterns so it is important to work through the earlier progressions as they will always be important in the design of your workouts. Proper rotation has to occur through the hip and NOT the lower back. Performed incorrectly the lower back could bear too much stress and because of the lack of movement in the base of the spine. The hip joint being a ball and socket possesses far more movement capabilities. Therefore, we must teach how to pivot and internally rotate one hip to allow the power hip to receive the weight and then produce force for the exercise. As eight time Powerlifting world champion, Ellen Stein describes this movement as, "putting out a cigarette." Yes, not the most health conscious cue, but something everyone can understand that one hip rotates inwards actively pressing weight through the ball of foot, while the other begins to hinge like we see in many of our accelerative training exercises such as cleans.

Often utilizing these rotational drills will not only increase your ability to be more injury resistant, or perform better in your everyday activities, but also tends to burn more calories as well! Below you can see an informal study that was done contrasting exercise complexity and calorie expenditure among two other popular forms of fat burning in functional training.

Because most training equipment doesn't even allow us this option exercise programs often miss this very important aspect of training. However, to properly introduce rotational Ultimate Sandbag™ training we need to take a progressive approach that we have used throughout our training DVRT™ system to ensure we see safe long-term success.

Because of the complexity of these movements we are going to focus on altering Range of Motion and Speed which will allow us to easily and incrementally progress through these progressions.

Foundational DVRT™ Rotation Drill: Rotational High Pulls

The High Pull is our starting point because the weight is close to our body decreasing the amount of force that the Ultimate Sandbag™ will act upon our body. Use the side of the knee as the starting point for the Rotational High Pull, do not try to over rotate as this will place more risk upon the low back. The side of the body that the Ultimate Sandbag™ is placed will be the working side. Hinge back into the lift with the opposing hip rotated so that the foot is pointing towards the working leg. Quickly extending the hips so the Ultimate Sandbag™ comes up and across the body with the elbows pointing up towards the sky. Do not pause in the middle, quickly rotate the working leg and the stance leg quickly plants and gets ready to absorb the force of the weight coming downwards.

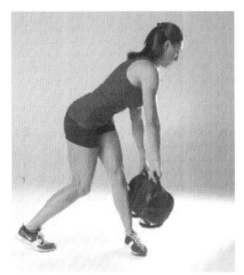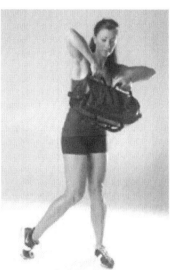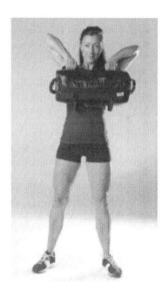

Instead of purely focusing on heavier weights in our rotational DVRT™ movements we can often simply work on trying to add more speed which gives the USB™ more leverage and perceived weight because of the added momentum. In this case if we move faster and faster in the Rotational High Pull and allow the weight to be projected higher upon our body we are able to eventually work into performing more challenging exercises such as the Half Moon Snatch.

The added challenge in DVRT™ drills like the Half Moon Snatch is that we have more weight to decelerate because of the higher point the weight reaches during the exercise. Yes, we produce more force and work harder on the way upwards, but many people are surprised how difficult the deceleration of the USB™ on the way down becomes. Therefore, it is VERY important to carefully work through being proficient with the Rotational High Pull and progressively work on pulling the USB™ to different points such as the chin, eyes, forehead, etc.

Advancing the Swing

The re-introduction of kettlebells back in the early 2000's also meant the revitalization of many old time lifts. One that specifically would become the most popular was the kettlebell swing. This exercise helped strengthen the low back and hips while being a tremendous way to get conditioning or "cardio" without a lot of space or impact upon the body. Unfortunately, the way the kettlebell swing is taught doesn't allow for advancing our movement skills and generally only lends itself to adding repetitions or weight which may not always be the best means of progressing.

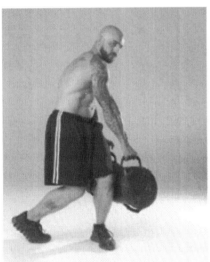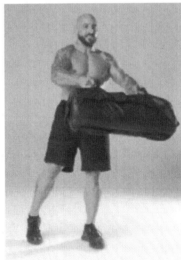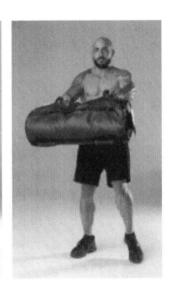

While the DVRT™ System does not try to replicate the kettlebell swing (there are other exercises in the DVRT™ that teach similar principles without swinging the USB™) we do have the ability to sophisticate the idea of the kettlebell swing. There are two primary DVRT™ drills that add amazing versatility and progression to the kettlebell swing and that is Shoveling and the Rotational Lunge. Very different in some respects you will find these either as the perfect compliment to your kettlebell swing training or advancing the movement.

Shoveling

Shoveling is recommend to be performed after one becomes proficient in movements like the Rotational High Pull and Half Moon Snatch. This is due to the fact we are going to create potentially great speed and have a longer lever arm than we do in the before mentioned drills. The Rotational Lunge is very misunderstood because of its name. The "rotational" component refers to the movement of the USB and not the lunge itself. In fact, the Rotational Lunge has little rotation to the body itself and is more of an anti-rotational lunge.

While the Rotational High Pull and Half Moon Snatch we are thinking of bringing the USB™ vertically "up" the body, Shoveling requires more of a projection of the USB™.

In order to perform Shoveling correctly we need to have a good understanding of how to absorb force and re-transmit it in the form of decelerating the USB™ as it comes back down to the side of our body. The arms are NOT "throwing" the USB™ rather an extension of the body trying to help maintain postural alignment while we perform Shoveling. The movement is performed solely by one hip extending and quickly rotating to prepare the body to absorb the downward momentum on the opposing side. When we receive the weight properly there is not definitive stop of the weight and the receiving hip quickly projects the USB™ again to the other side making a smooth back and forth arching pattern.

Shoveling can be progressed by changing speed. Not going as fast or producing as much force we can keep the USB™ from swinging as far from the body decreasing the amount of force we have to then absorb. This is a good progression for those that are trying to learn the movement or beginners.

Rotational Lunge

Possibly one of the favorite and most unusual DVRT™ drills. The Rotational Lunge is unique in the fact we have the body in moving one plane of motion while the USB™ is moving and pulling in the other two planes. So not only is the body having to work to lunge back and forth but to resist the pull of the USB™ side to side.

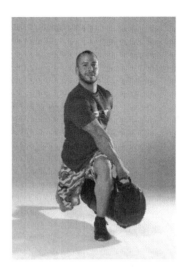

Similar to the kettlebell swing and Shoveling, we see a projection of the weight out in front of the body. However, now we are trying to resist rotation of the body and we are working from a more unstable stance which greatly increases the intensity of the exercise even at lighter USB™ weights.

While the ultimate goal is to try to project the USB™ to chest height while not compromising the reverse lunge we can begin at smaller increments of movement so more people can appreciate the power of this drill.

- Progression 1: Rotate Slowly Only to the Same Side

- Progression 2: Rotate Slowly Alternating Side

- Progression 3: Begin to Add Speed by Aiming to Reach
  Different Projection Heights on the Body

Putting It All Together

The DVRT™ program contains over 300 exercises which means no shortage of variations or progressions. Yet, performing the exercises are just part of the equation. Learning how to piece the exercises along with other training variables produces something extraordinary. This means we have to have a plan and philosophy of how to integrate these exercises and programs effectively and simply.

How does DVRT Training Compare?

Trained Female #1

Training Variable	Kettlebell Two Handed Swings	Rotational Lunge	Battling Ropes Both Arms Up & Down
Average Heart Rate	121	141	125
Calories	53	83	45
Time	5 min 37 seconds	6 min 43 seconds	4 min 29 seconds
Weight	35 pounds	17 pounds	50 foot 1.5 inch
Repetitions	100	50 each side	200

Trained Male #1

Training Variable	Kettlebell Two Handed Swings	Rotational Lunge	Battling Ropes Both Arms Up & Down
Average Heart Rate	154	170	153
Calories	83	98	82
Time	5 min 46 seconds	5 min 48 seconds	5 min 44 seconds
Weight	70 pounds	33 pounds	50 foot 1.5 inch rope
Repetitions	100	42 each side	300

Which and How Many

Probably the most common question anyone has about any fitness program is which and how many exercises to place within a program. The answer is not necessarily an easy one. It depends on how many days a week you train, the level of complexity of the movements, and your own current fitness level.

Here are some general guidelines and then we will provide some specific situations.

- The more frequently you train the less number of exercises you perform.

- The more complex the movements, the less number of exercises you perform.

- The greater perceived intensity of the exercise the less number of exercises you will perform.

While these are good guidelines it is more helpful if we look at some practical examples. For most people anywhere from three to four days of training in the DVRT™ system will be optimal. Especially starting with three is not a bad idea because the recovery of this unique stress may vary quite a bit depending upon the individual.

Once you determined how many days a week we can then consider the number of exercises. Three to eight exercises can be used per workout, however, if you wish to perform more exercises per workout varying the intensity of the movements is important in keeping balance and avoiding overtraining. How to combine these movements will be discussed shortly to give some ideas of how to create highly effective programs.

Which Exercises Should I Perform?

Often it is very sad to hear that people become bored or stale with their fitness programs. In the DVRT™ System that should never happen. There are great progressions and variety built into every exercise. Coming up we will discuss how to also alter repetitions and sets, but now lets look at which exercises you should select.

The beauty in understanding the basics of creating effective programs is that you have so many more options that most people believe. If we first look at most functional movement patterns we will see a great number of choices in just movements.

Functional Movement Patterns:

- Squatting
- Stepping (Lunging and Step-ups)
- Hip Hinging
- Vertical Pressing
- Vertical Pulling
- Horizontal Pressing
- Horizontal Pulling
- Rotation of Body
- Anti-Rotation
- Flexion of the Trunk
- Anti-Flexion
- Jumping
- Running

From this list alone we should never have a reason to plateau or feel unfulfilled by our training. However, it also means we don't have to be so random that we have no plan either. Striking balance gives the optimal training environment.

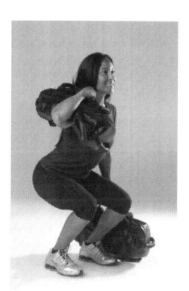

Here is an example of how a few exercises in the DVRT™ system crossover in the above list. For example a Shoulder Squat is both squatting and anti-rotation.

Example Workout 1

Exercise	Pattern	Sets	Reps	Rest
Reverse Shoulder Lunge	Stepping/Lower Body Pull/Anti-Rotation	3-4	6-8 each leg	45 seconds
Clean and Press	Lower Body Pull/ Vertical Pressing/ Vertical Pulling/ Anti-Flexion	3-4	5-7	45 seconds
Bear Hug Squat	Squatting/ Horizontal Pulling	2-3	10-12	45 seconds
Bent-over Rowing	Horizontal Pulling/Anti-Flexion	2-3	10-12	45 seconds
Around the World	Rotation/Anti-Flexion	2-3	30 Seconds Each Direction	45 seconds

With the above example we should feel more confident that we don't have to perform a large number of exercises to get an amazingly effective workout. This is also the reason that we need to plan out workouts so that we don't have overly redundant training that both causes boredom and plateaus. Therefore, if we were to perform three days a week of workouts the other day may see the following plan.

Example Workout 2

Exercise	Pattern	Sets	Reps	Rest
Shoulder to Shoulder Squat	Squat/Anti-Rotation/Lower Body Pull	3-4	4-5 Each Side	45 seconds
Push-ups	Horizontal Pushing/Anti-Flexion	3-4	10-15	45 seconds
Lateral Lunge High Pull	Stepping/Lower Body Pull	2-3	8-10 Per Side	45 seconds
Pull-ups	Vertical Pulling/Anti-Flexion	2-3	6-8	45 seconds
Shoulder Get-up	Rotation/Anti-Flexion/Lower Body Pull	2-3	5 each side	45 seconds

Example Workout 3

Exercise	Pattern	Sets	Reps	Rest
Rotational Lunge Clean	Stepping/Lower Body Pull/ Rotation/Anti-Rotation	3-4	8-10 Each Leg	45 seconds
Half Knee Shoulder to Shoulder Press	Vertical Pushing/ Vertical Pulling/ Anti-Rotation	3-4	6-8 Each Side	45 seconds
Staggered Bear Hug Squat	Squatting/ Horizontal Pulling	2-3	10-12 Each Side	45 seconds
Push-up Plank to Lateral Drag	Horizontal Pulling/Anti-Flexion/Anti-Rotation	2-3	5-6 Each Side	45 seconds
Rotational Chops	Rotation/Anti-Flexion	2-3	10-15 Each Side	45 seconds

It is important to note that not all exercises and movements are equal. Some Ultimate Sandbag™ drills are more fluid such as Rotational Lunges, Shoveling, and Around the Worlds. Others are based upon more of a tension model. This can vary in how the tension is applied but focuses around some foundational movements such as squats, overhead pressing, cleans, rows, lunging, etc.

Not all patterns are going to be emphasized in the same manner. One great example is the de-emphasis of trunk flexion types of movements because of the large amount of sitting and crunches that our culture is prone to performing. Rather you will see a de-emphasis of trunk flexion drills and more exercises that are teaching how to resist trunk flexion. Many of these such drills include those that have the Ultimate Sandbag™ in the Zercher position.

In the case of rotational drills we could argue that people have to learn how to resist rotation and control those forces before they start performing more complex drills. However, the idea of learning how to resist rotation does serve as a useful format for more successful training programs. For example because it is not just whether not we squat that is of concern, but how the Ultimate Sandbag™ weight is being applied such as the Shoulder position which teaches a lot of anti-rotation skills.

Therefore, it is very important to address which Ultimate Sandbags™ weights and holding positions we should be prioritizing as this will equally impact the training program. Below I have provided recommendations, and of course, these are just recommendations and can be tailored to the individual.

Size of Ultimate Sandbag™	Weight	Training Goal
Power Ultimate Sandbag™	10-20 Pounds	-Movement oriented drills that involve more dynamic motion. -Rotational based drills -Stabilization exercises
Power Ultimate Sandbag™	20-35 Pounds	-Hybrid exercises: those that involve multiple large movements -Strength based exercises such as squats, cleans, rows, and presses
Strength Ultimate Sandbag™	20-35 Pounds (lighter filling implements such as rice may be used to give dimension while keeping weight down)	-Progressing to more unstable training. -Working with larger dimensions. -Increasing intensity of exercises. -Can be used as corrective tool for beginner to intermediate individuals.

Size of Ultimate Sandbag™	Weight	Training Goal
Strength Ultimate Sandbag™	40-80 Pounds	-Using load as more of a focus for strength lifts such as squats, rows, cleans, and presses -Great for blend of strength development and conditioning.
Burly Ultimate Sandbag™	50-80 Pounds (lighter filling implements such as rice may be used to give dimension while keeping weight down)	-Focus on using dimension to create more of a challenge than purely weight. -Can be used as a corrective tool for more advanced lifters.
Burly Ultimate Sandbag™	85-120 Pounds	-The most challenging level of instability, weight, and dimension. -More advanced lifters and athletes.
Burly Ultimate Sandbag™	120-180 Pounds	-For advanced athletes focusing upon strength based lifts and strongman type of exercises such as carries.

Establishing the size of Ultimate Sandbag™ is part of the equation, when we assign the exercises we also want to understand the progressions of the holding positions. Understanding the progressions allow you to greatly vary the movements without having to change the actual weight of the Ultimate Sandbag™. Although we are not focusing on changing the weight of the Ultimate Sandbag™ it does not mean that these exercises will be easy, in fact, sometimes changing the holding position of the Ultimate Sandbag™ seems significantly more difficult than adding weight. There are up to 12 different holding positions but the majority of your training will be focused on four different variations (overhead itself offers three different variations to challenge the body)!

Holding Position 1: Bear Hug

Holding Position 2: Zercher Position

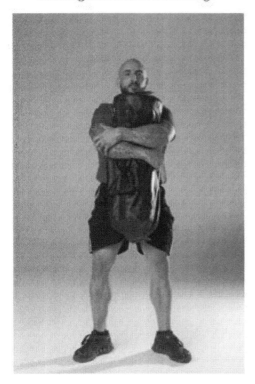

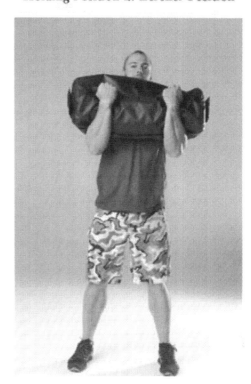

Holding Position 3: Shoulder (when moving to single leg drills placing the Ultimate Sandbag on the opposite side of the stance leg is easier than the same side)

Opposite Side

Same Side

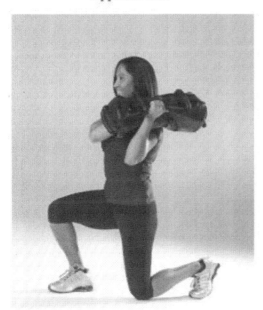

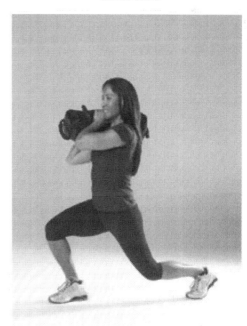

Overhead Offers Three Variations:

Option 1: Snatch Grip

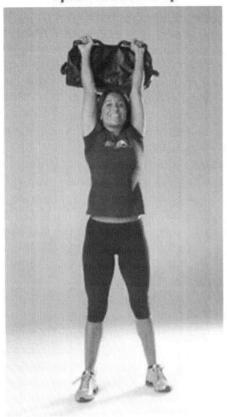

Option 2: Neutral Grip

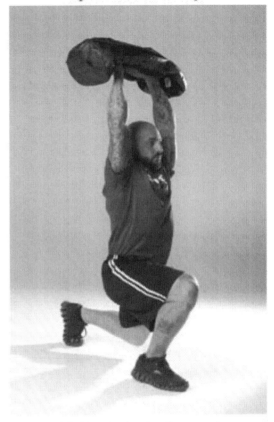

Option 3: Mid-Grip

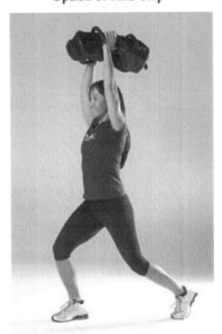

*Option 4: Single Arm Only

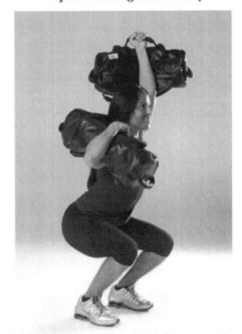

*Recommended with smaller Ultimate Sandbags

The Workouts

Now it is time to discuss the various workouts you can immediately implement and start to benefit from right now! Ultimate Sandbags™ lend themselves best to two types of training, Ladders and Intervals.

Ladders:

Ladders are a valuable training method that allows us to do a good amount of work at a high level. They also provide us the opportunity to use heavier loads or more complex movements that might not be possible with traditional repetition schemes.

For example, it would be common to have someone perform 15 repetitions of an exercise. However, that means we probably are going to have low complexity and low load, the more we can raise either of these components the faster we can see changes to our fitness goals.

Instead of that set of 15 repetitions we could perform a series of 1/2/3/4/5 or 5/4/3/2/1. Since ladders are typically supersetted (alternated between two movements) a better scenario may look like the following:

Bear Hug Squat: 5/4/3/2/1

Pull-ups: 1/2/3/4/5

This means that you would perform 5 repetitions of Bear Hug Squats immediately followed by 1 Pull-up, immediately back to 4 Bear Hug Squats followed right away by 2 Pull-ups. You would continue the ladder until all the repetitions were completed and then follow the prescribed rest interval. This equals one set of a ladder and is often more intense than standard high repetition work.

Intervals:

An interval is a specific amount of time that one performs the exercise. Common intervals are anywhere from 15 seconds up to a minute. If we have a work interval we must also have a rest interval. Most common rest intervals can be from 15 seconds up to 2 minutes. When we refer to the work time and rest time we call that work to rest ratio.

Many people begin too aggressively both on the amount of time they are working and making the rest time too short.

It is not uncommon to see people try to perform 1:1 work to ratios. A popular example is a 30 seconds of work followed by 30 seconds of rest. While such a time frame may not sound very difficult the truth is that a 1:1 ratio is quite intense and especially people new to such training are better served with a 1:2 work to rest. This would change our above example to 30 seconds of work followed by 60 seconds of rest. Instead of adding weight to our exercise we would decrease our rest interval and/or increase our work time.

Having the goal of a 1:1 work to rest ratio is a solid level of fitness and a great goal to set forth. However, advanced training can take advantage of a NEGATIVE work to rest ratio. This would be mean performing 30 seconds of work and only giving yourself 15 or 20 seconds of rest. Such training is VERY intense and should be saved for more intense training programs.

Can I Just Use Standard Sets and Reps?

Of course you can apply your standard sets and reps such as 3 sets of 10, however, having standards to progress are key. Since Ultimate Sandbags™ do not lend themselves to 5 pound increment increases in weight relying on such protocols may be quite challenging. Below are several examples of how you can blend these methods together.

Beginner Workout 1

Exercise	Sets	Repetitions	Rest Interval
A1. Bear Hug Squats	2 Rounds	5/4/3/2/1	0
A2. Bent-Over Row	2 Rounds	10/8/6/4/2	120 Seconds
B1. Shoulder Forward Lunge Alternating Legs	2 Sets	20 Seconds	40 Seconds
B2. Shoulder to Shoulder Press	2 Sets	20 Seconds	40 Seconds
C1. Push-up Hold	2 Sets	30 Seconds	30 Seconds
C2. Biceps Curl	2 Sets	8-12 Repetitions	30 Seconds

Bent-Over Row   **Shoulder Forward Lunge**   **Biceps Curl**

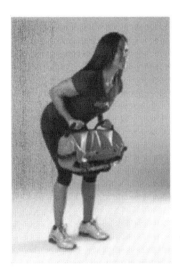
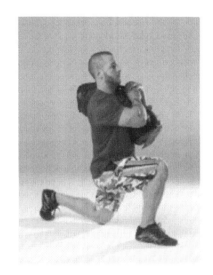
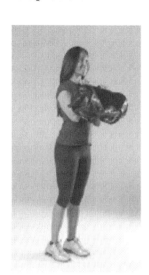

What makes for a "beginner workout?" When someone first tries Ultimate Sandbag™ they can be surprised how many "new" muscles are targeted. Therefore the first variable we work with is the amount of work we perform. That is why you will see a build up on foundational movements and performing less sets. Over time we could use the same program, but slightly increase the amount of sets used in the workout.

These workouts also start us with more stable body and Ultimate Sandbag™ holding positions and postures. Over time we can simply change the way we hold or position the Ultimate Sandbag™. For example we can change Bear Hug Squats to Bear Hug Staggered Squats or Zercher Squats depending upon our training goal. We can change the Bent-Over Row simply by switching the handles we use or if we go to a more unstable body position such as staggered or single leg.

Considerations of Beginner Workouts

This program is designed to be a three days a week program, a rest day should be utilized between workouts. This offers a great opportunity to learn the foundations of many of the USB™ workouts and recover from the training.

A "beginner" workout does not imply that these movements cannot be optimized by other levels of fitness. We can change the amount of work, the weight, speed of movement, and position of the USB™ to add increased challenges to any of these movements. For example, during workout 2 we can increase the work time from 20 seconds to 30 seconds and/or decrease the rest interval from 40 seconds to 30 down to 20 seconds.

Track your progress using the workouts listed previously, as a guide. This can be a six to eight week program depending on how fast you adapt.

Beginner Workout 2

Exercise	Sets	Repetitions	Rest Interval
A1. Power Clean to Overhead Press	2	20 Seconds	40 Seconds
A2. Two Point Row	2	20 Seconds	40 Seconds
A3. Zercher Step-ups	2	20 Seconds	40 Seconds
A4. Side Plank	2	20 Seconds Each Side	40 Seconds
A5. Bear Hug Goodmornings	2	20 Seconds	40 Seconds
A6. Lying Floor Press	2	20 Seconds	40 Seconds

Two Point Row

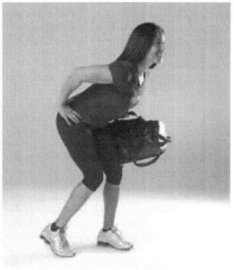

Zercher Step-up

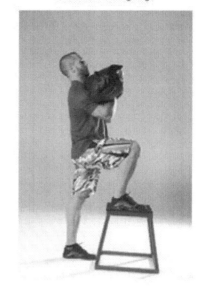

Bear Hug Goodmornings

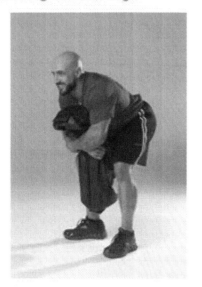

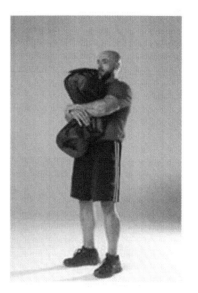

Lying Floor Press

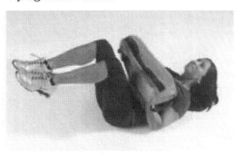

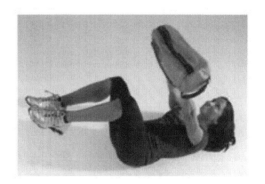

Beginner Workout 3

Exercise	Sets	Repetitions	Rest Intervals
A1. Bear Hug Lateral Lunge	2	8-10 each side	60 Seconds
A2. Half Kneeling Shoulder to Shoulder Press	2	10-12 per side	60 Seconds
A3. Single Leg Deadlift: Bilateral Grip	2	8-10 each side	60 Seconds
A4. Shoulder Get-up to Bridge	2	5-6 each side	60 Seconds
A5. Golf Swing	2	15-20 per side	60 Seconds

Bear Hug Lateral Lunge   **Half Kneeling Shoulder to Shoulder Press**

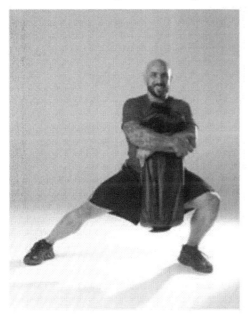
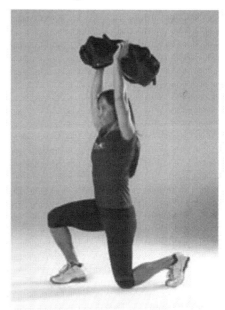

Single Leg Deadlift Bilateral Grip

Golf Swing: Phase 1

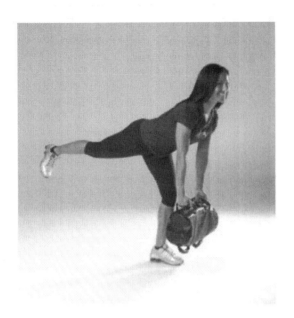

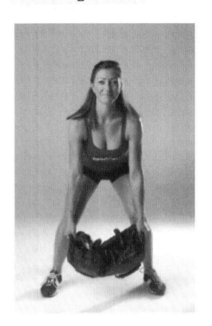

Golf Swing: Phase 2

Golf Swing: Phase 3
(Immediately Swing in Opposing Direction)

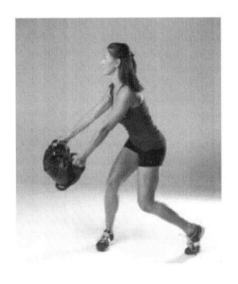

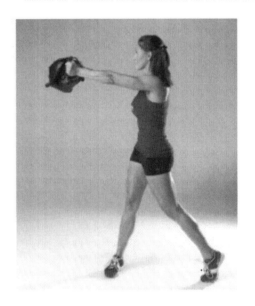

Shoulder Get-up to Bridge:
Phase 1   **Phase 2**

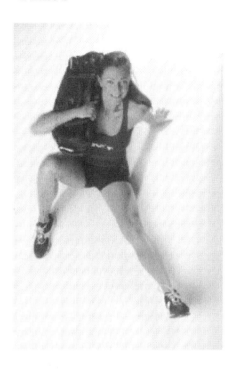   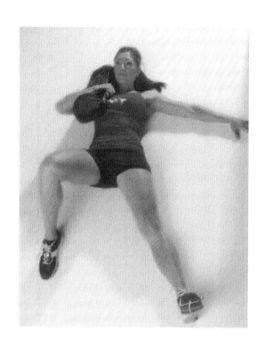

Phase 3

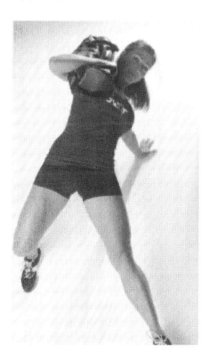

Intro to the Intermediate Workouts

Intermediate Workout 1

Exercise	Sets	Repetitions	Rest Intervals
A1. Zercher Staggered Squats	3-4 Rounds	10/8/6/4/2	0
A2. Kneeling Presses	3-4 Rounds	10/8/6/4/2	60-120 Seconds
B1. Rotational Lunge	2-3	30-40 Seconds	40 Seconds
B2. Plank Forward/ Back Drag	2-3	5-8 each Direction	40 Seconds
B3. Grip Curls	2-3	10-12	40 Seconds

Rotational Lunge

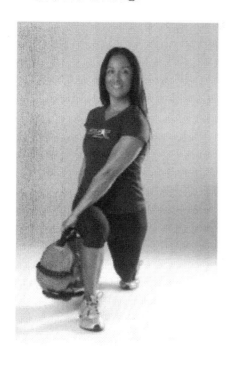

Plank Drag Forward and Back

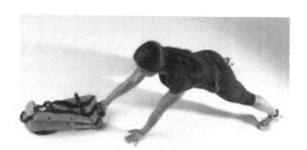

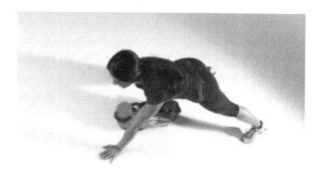

Grip Curls

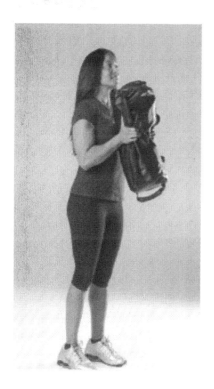 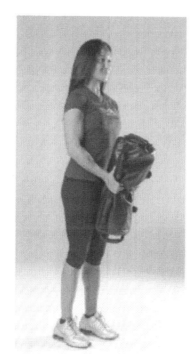

Intermediate Workout 2

Exercise	Sets	Repetitions	Rest Intervals
A1. Lunge to Overhead Press	2-4 Rounds	30-40 Seconds	40-60 Seconds
A2. Supinated Rows	2-4 Rounds	30-40 Seconds	40-60 Seconds
A3. Rotational High Pull	2-4 Rounds	30-40 Seconds	40-60 Seconds
A5. Side to Side Floor Press	2-4 Rounds	30-40 Seconds	40-60 Seconds

Lunge to Overhead Press

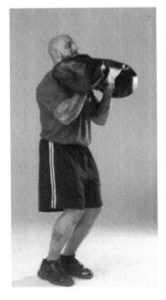 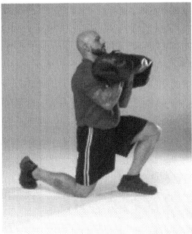 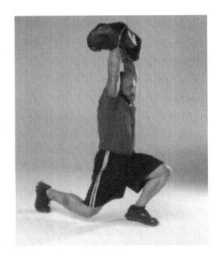

Supinated Rows

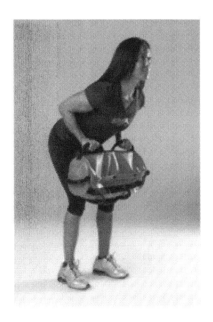

Rotational High Pull Phase 1:

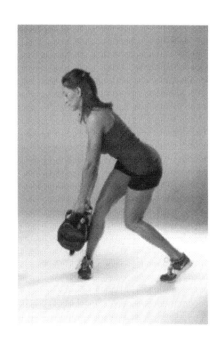

Rotational High Pull Phase 2:

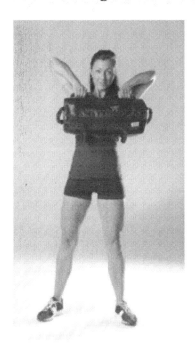

Floor Press Side to Side

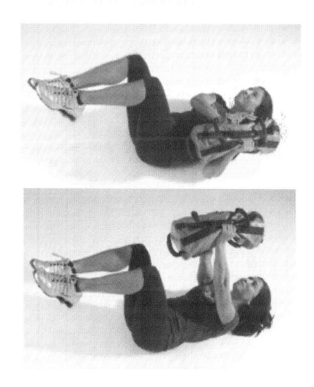

Intermediate Workout 3

Exercise	Sets	Repetitions	Rest Intervals
A1. Pronated Rows to Power Snatch	3-4	2 Rows/1 Snatch=5 Rounds	60 Seconds
A2. Shoulder Squat	3-4	5-6 Switch Sides	60 Seconds
B1. Shoulder Get-up	2-3	5-6 Each side	30-45 Seconds
B2. Around the World	2-3	20-30 Seconds Each Side	30-45 Seconds
B3. Plank Walk-up To Push-up	2-3	10-15	30-45 Seconds

Pronated Rows to Power Snatch

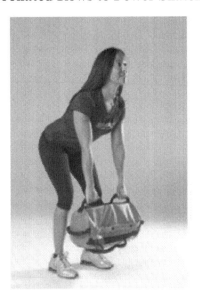 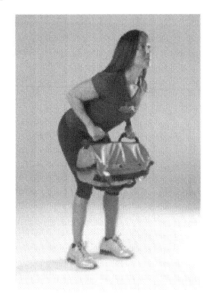 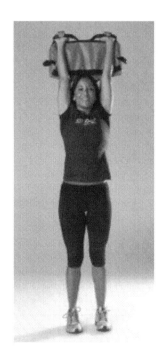

Around The World

Phase 1   Phase 2   Phase 3

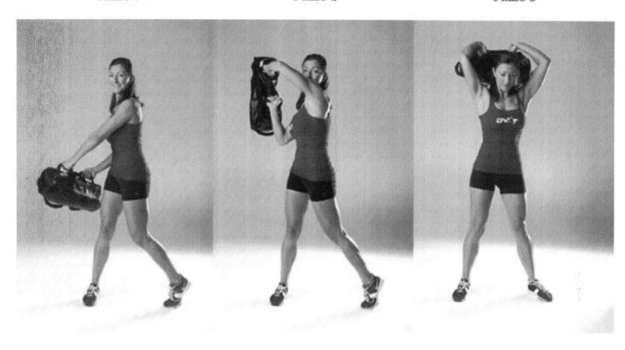

Phase 4   Phase 5   Phase 6

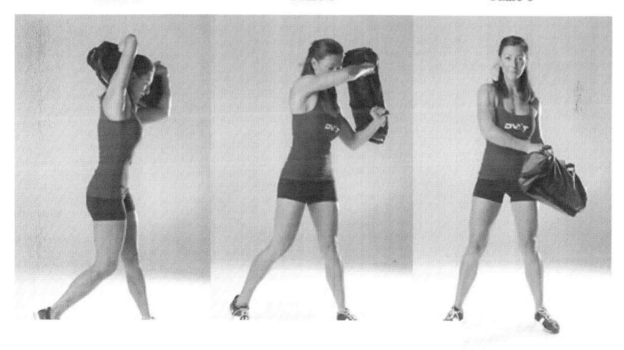

Intro to Advanced Workouts

Advanced Workout 1

Exercise	Sets	Repetitions	Rest Intervals
A1. Rotational Snatch to Overhead Lunge	3-4	5/4/3/2/1 Perform Alternating Sets with A2. then Switch the Lead Side	0
A2. One Legged Rows-Same Side Dumbbell Style	3-4	12/8/6/4/2 Switch Legs with Each Series, Switch Which Leg You Begin	60 Seconds
B1. Shoulder Lateral Lunge	3-4	10-12 Each Side	40-60 Seconds
B2. Lateral Plank Drag	3-4	5-8 Per Side, Slow Temps	40-60 Seconds
B3. Bear Hug Walks	3-4	Walk in Bear Hug Position for 30-60 Seconds	40-60 Seconds

Rotational Snatch to Overhead Lunge

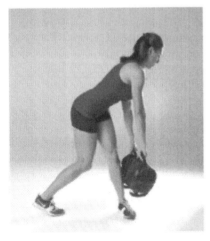 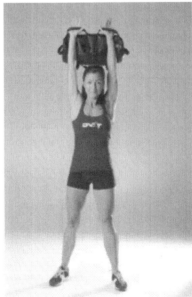 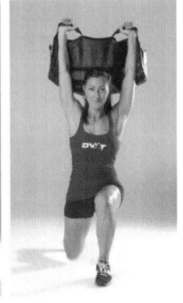

One Legged Rows-Same Side Dumbbell Style   **Shoulder Lateral Lunge-On Outside**

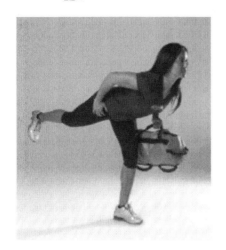   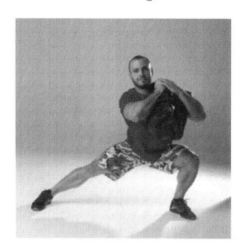

Lateral Plank Drag

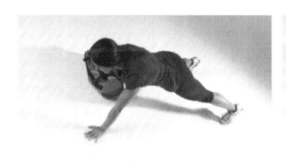   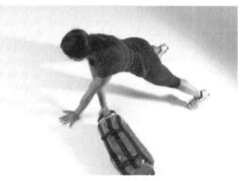

Bent Over Row Grip Style

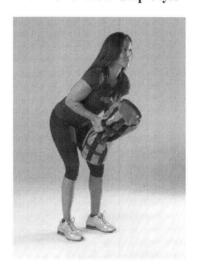

Advanced Workout 2

Exercise	Sets	Repetitions	Rest Intervals
A1. Rotational Lunges-Get USB to Chest Height	3-4	40 Seconds	20 Seconds
A2. Bent-Over Row: Grip Style (Grip the Middle of the USB)	3-4	40 Seconds	20 Seconds
A3. Shoulder to Shoulder Thruster	3-4	40 Seconds	20 Seconds
A4. Shoulder Leg Threading	3-4	40 Seconds Each Side	20 Seconds
A5. Front Planks with One Leg Elevated	3-4	40 Seconds	20 Seconds

Bent-over Row Grip Style

During the progressions of both the Intermediate and Advanced Ultimate Sandbag™ workouts we can see an evolution to more complex patterns. This can come in the form of moving into staggered Zercher squats in the Intermediate program to more single leg and speed variables in the Advanced workouts.

The important concept to take note is that any of these movements and progressions and regressions that can allow us to utilize components with any fitness level. Whether that is changing the amount of repetitions and sets you perform to altering speed and leverage. For example in the rotational snatch to overhead lunge we could substitute a rotational clean to zercher lunge to reduce leverage or we can take it back a step to staggered stance clean to forward lunge. Having so many options ensures you always can have success!

Shoulder to Shoulder Thruster

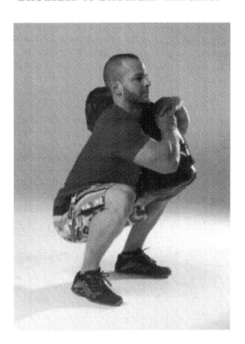 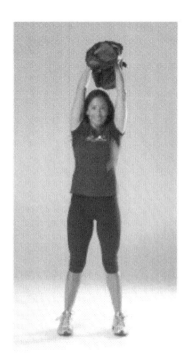

Leg Threading

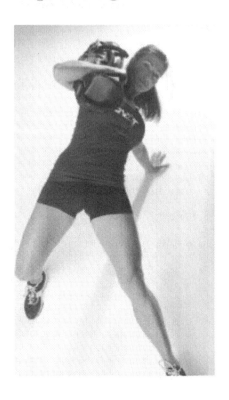 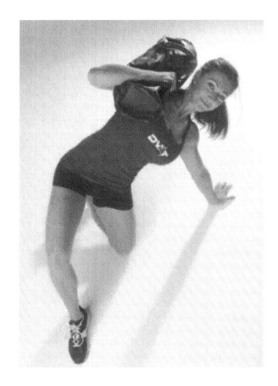

Advanced Workout 3

Exercise	Sets	Repetitions	Rest Intervals
A1. Staggered Clean-Zercher Squat-Press	5	5 each side	60 Seconds
B1. Pull-ups	3-4	6-8	45 Seconds
B2. Half Moon Snatch	3-4	10-12 per side	45 Seconds
B3. Side Plank Rows	3-4	10-15 per side	45 Seconds
B4. Overhead Crossover Lunge	3-4	8-10 per side	45 Seconds

Staggered Clean-Squat Press

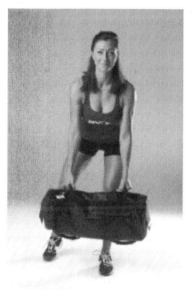 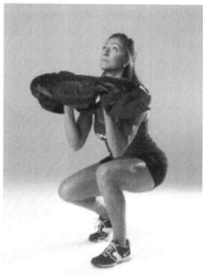 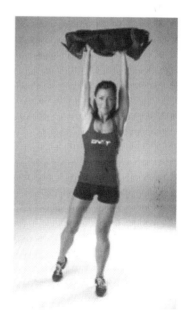

Half Moon Snatch

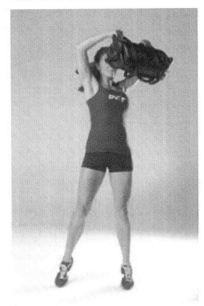 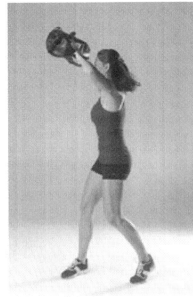 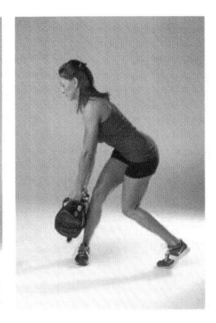

Side Plank Rows

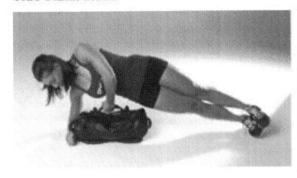 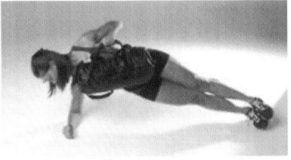

The term "Advanced" in the DVRT™ program goes far beyond just using heavier weights. You will see a great deal of complexity of movement used to challenge your level of fitness. Complexity can offer the perfect balance of strength, conditioning, athleticism and mobility.

Overhead Crossover Lunge

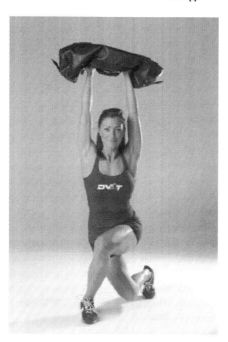

During the advanced workout series you are seeing more challenging body positions and the implementation of more complexes. A complex refers to several movements being used within one exercise. This is done for several benefits:

• Increased Number of Muscles Used

• Greater Energy Expenditure

• More Work in Less Time!

Complexity also allows us to use one Ultimate Sandbag™ if we wish, or keeps the number of Ultimate Sandbags™ down to a minimum. With almost every other weight training program you have to accumulate more and more equipment as you progress. Not necessarily true with the DVRT™ that actually continually demonstrates the value of Ultimate Sandbags™ that you may have believed you "out grew."

Just because we are hitting the advanced phase doesn't mean that we have to increase the number of workouts either! That is one of the major mistakes when people progress through training programs, the belief that MORE is better! Because we are raising the intensity whether it is from the complexity of the actual exercises or extending work intervals or adding in more combination exercises, monitoring your success with a three day a week program is far wiser!

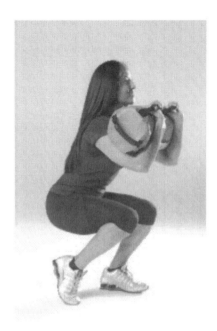

How do you know? It all goes back to goal setting. One of the biggest values of our DVRT™ system is the fact we are not promoting a program to get you better at sandbag training! No, we want the Ultimate Sandbag™ to be a solution to your fitness needs. Each individual is going to be different, but the beauty of the DVRT™ is the fact it is so flexible that it can mold itself to any fitness goal.

Common Questions in Ultimate Sandbag™ Training

Q: Should my Ultimate Sandbag™ be shifting and moving? As I go heavier it shifts less, is that normal?

A: There is the unfortunate belief that the primary benefit of sandbag training is this drastic shifting of weight inside. The truth is that instability should be as progressive as weight or performing more repetitions. However, we tried to do a lot of the problem solving and programming for you.

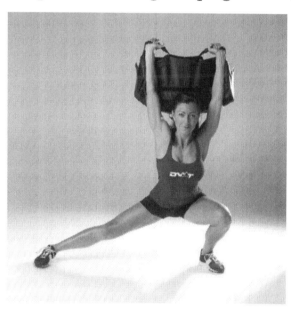

That means that we recommend the Power Ultimate Sandbag™ for beginning women and Strength Ultimate Sandbag™ for beginning men. Why? Because at lighter weights you will have a more unstable Ultimate Sandbag™, however, in designing this system we therefore also controlled the dimension. So we didn't want people being introduced to Ultimate Sandbags™ to have to deal with an unreasonable level of instability, just the RIGHT amount to getting a great training experience.

As the Ultimate Sandbag™ becomes heavier because you are getting stronger you are introduce to dealing with heavier weights by reducing the instability. You see when we increase one variable, we have to gently decrease the other so that we provide a more progressive system rather than a giant SHOCK that both high levels of weight and instability would provide. For many people, the progression lies something in the following:

- Unstable Smaller Ultimate Sandbag™ > More Stable But Heavier Smaller Ultimate Sandbag™ >
- Same Weight, but Larger Ultimate Sandbag™ which increases the instability again.

Just as with everything we describe and recommend in the DVRT™ program there should be progressions to all these variables and shifting weight is an important one!

Q: When I want to make an exercise or workout more challenging should I use a heavier Ultimate Sandbag™ or change something else?

A: Great question and it really depends on your goals and the number of Ultimate Sandbags™ that you have available to use in your training. Let's examine a few examples.

I'll admit if you have two Ultimate Sandbags™ you have more options than if you have one. Yet, it doesn't mean you don't have a TON of different ways that you can still progress through different exercises or workouts.

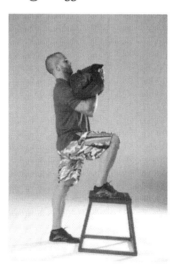

If the goal is primarily fat or weight loss then load doesn't have to be quite as big of a concern. Simply by changing the position of the Ultimate Sandbag™ and/or body position you can definitely change the level of exercise. Some of these positional changes may seem more subtle than others. For example, moving from the Bear Hug position to the Zercher Position tends to be an easier transition than from the Zercher position to the Shoulder position because the distance the weight actually moves is less and the stability goes from being primarily in front of the body to the side.

Others will find changing body positions to be potentially more of a challenge. Moving from a more stable squatting position to some of the single leg stance exercises can be a significant increase in perceived challenge of the exercise. That is why in both scenarios we recommend small progressive changes and follow this progression:

Stable Body Position (i.e. Squats, Bilateral Power Lifts, Bilateral Pressing/Rowing Exercises)->Stable Load Position (i.e. Bear Hug Position)->Stable Body Position->Unstable Load Position (i.e. Moving Towards Shoulder and Overhead Positions)->Unstable Body Position (i.e. Staggered or Split Stances)->Stable Load Position->Unstable Body & Unstable Load Positions

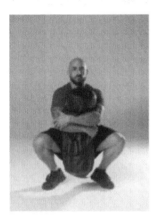 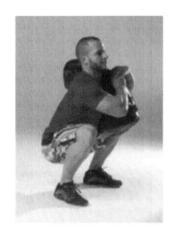 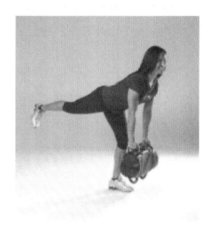

Viewing exercise this way may be very different for most people. That is ok! Once you start breaking down the movements in such a manner you begin to see that you have way more options than you may have ever considered in making your workouts diverse, fun, and most importantly, highly effective.

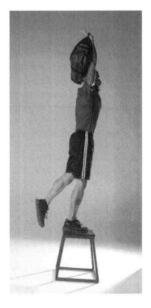

Unstable Body & Unstable Load

For those that are striving for fat loss you will find that working through such progressions makes your investment of one Ultimate Sandbag™ feel as though you have a full gym at your finger tips! Unlike many other fat loss programs these just don't make you sweat! You will find that you develop functional strength and muscle so that you will keep your metabolism jump started for hours after you are done training.

Probably one of the most surprising benefits to people that use the Ultimate Sandbag™ as a means to shred fat is the fact that they don't beat up their bodies in the same way they would performing a host of other fitness programs. This is due to the much lower impact that Ultimate Sandbag™ training provides, the lack of repetitive movements, and how your stabilizers are strengthened to give long-term support to your joints.

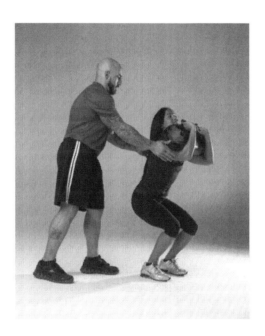

Let's face it, very few people ever mind get leaner, so even if your goal is strength and performance you can use a similar model of progression. One of the more unique aspects of Ultimate Sandbag™ training is the fact that it blends the best of Olympic lifting, Powerlifting, Strongman, and Functional Fitness to provide such an incredibly unique training experience that often people have a hard time believing it can do all that I am promising until they start performing the workout programs.

So does that mean you can't go heavier? For those that might have a more serious devotion to strength and performance goals you can use the same progressions but vary the training schedule that you perform or how you organize the exercises in the workouts.

Training Schedule for DVRT™ Strength Emphasis

Mon.	Tues.	Wed.	Thurs.	Fri.	Sat.	Sun.
Stable Strength Lower Body Exercise Emphasis Unstable Body & Load Position Upper Body	Stable Body & Load Position Upper Body Emphasis Unstable Body & Load Position Lower Body	Active Recovery (Yoga, Stretch, etc.)	Unstable Body Position & Stable Load Position Lower Body Emphasis Unstable Body & Unstable Load Position Upper Body Emphasis	Unstable Body Position & Stable Load Position Upper Body Emphasis Lower Body & Unstable Load Position Lower Body Emphasis	Active Recovery	Off

What are Some Examples?

Mon.	Tues.	Wed.	Thurs.	Fri.	Sat.	Sun.
1. Zercher Squat 2. Half Kneeling Shoulder to Shoulder Press	1. Clean and Press 2. Rotational Lunge	Active Recovery	1. Bear Hug Staggered Stance Squat 2. One Leg Pronated Row	1. Staggered Overhead Press 2. Off-set Single Leg Deadlift	Active Recovery	Off

Q: Coach Henkin, I love to have a "finisher" to my workouts, what do you recommend? I like carrying Ultimate Sandbags™ what do you think?

A: For those that are unfamiliar, a "finisher" is just what the name implies. It is a single exercise that is usually done to train more of a conditioning component of fitness and hit the whole body at once, somewhat symbolizing the end of the workout because no more productive work could be performed. So, is a finisher necessary? Not really, you don't HAVE to perform one, in fact, most people will feel as though they have absolutely no need or desire once they go through some of the workout programs listed in this book.

However, if you do wish to perform a finisher, Ultimate Sandbag™ carries can be great. Many coaches have become fascinated with Farmer's Walks (an exercise where you carry weights down by your side), yet, I believe Ultimate Sandbag™ carries offer far more variety and benefits.

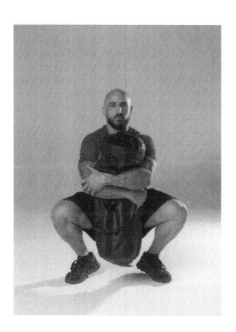

Walking with Ultimate Sandbags™ in any of the positions (Bear Hug, Zercher, Shoulder, Overhead, X-Patterns) are phenomenal ways to progressively challenge the strength and stability of the entire body. The advantage of Ultimate Sandbag™ walking drills is that the load is placed higher in relationship to the body than Farmer's Walks, that means less weight can actually be used to stress the body just as much, if not more!

We could also make the argument that Ultimate Sandbag™ carries actually hit more muscles than Farmer's Walks and doesn't have the potential to work on important stability concepts either, let me explain.

Heavy Farmer's Walks place a lot of strain on the biceps and the tendon because they are trying to resist the arm from being hyperextended. That is why in many professional Strongman contests, it is not uncommon for athletes to tear or rupture their biceps tendon. With the Ultimate Sandbag™ Bear Hug or Zercher Positions the arms are being taxed in a more flexed position. Because the muscles are working so hard to maintain the contraction, most people feel the arms far more taxed than in the Farmer's Walk. Additionally, because of this flexed position the biceps and tendon are not nearly at the risk to get injured.

Some will say that Farmer's Walks work the postural muscles of the upper back to a significant degree. They do! However, because of the placement of load (down by the hips) it takes far more relative weight to stress that area than if you performed the same work via the Bear Hug and Zercher carrying positions. Most importantly changing the body's center of gravity by changing the placement of the Ultimate Sandbag™ you get increased work of the core.

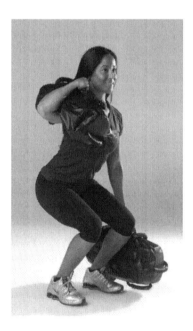

"But you can perform one-arm Farmer's Walks to challenge core stability." True, but if you really want to get a more accurate or better demonstration of core stability during carrying try maintaining your posture while performing Shoulder or various Overhead carries. The Ultimate Sandbag Shoulder Position may look to be a simple sagittal pain movement but it is far more complex because of the effort involved in not allowing the weight to cause rotation or side bending to occur. Just a little bit goes a long way!

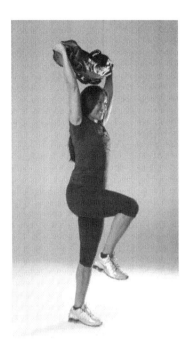

Finally, we have two different means of going overhead. In the Snatch position we can introduce the hardest leverage point to Ultimate Sandbag™ carries and emphasis "opening up" the thoracic spine and shoulders while also training the upper back and core muscles. Transitioning to the Overhead position on the fists makes us have to balance not only the position of the weight Overhead, but the instability of the Ultimate Sandbag™ as well. Want the to bring all these benefits together? Try some X-Patterns and see how much your whole body can be torched by some lighter Ultimate Sandbags™.

How should you introduce Ultimate Sandbag™ carries? Just in the same manner as all our Ultimate Sandbag™ exercises. Begin with the most stable position and work on building up time. Therefore performing a few sets of 30 seconds of walking and once you can get to 2 minutes you can change the holding position.

Q: I don't understand why the Power Ultimate Sandbag™ has handles on the side and the larger ones have these strange flaps?

A: This difference often confuses a lot of people as far as the intent of some of the features on the Ultimate Sandbag™. Understanding biomechanics of the body, you would see lifting the smallest of our Ultimate Sandbags™ (the Power USB) by the top parallel handles would create to narrow of a pressing base for the shoulders. In order to put the shoulders in the right position we placed side handles in order to allow people to press from a healthier shoulder position.

The reverse is almost true of our Strength and Burly USBs. Because they become longer in dimension, trying to put the Ultimate Sandbag™ overhead while grabbing the flaps places the shoulders in a compromised position. That is why it is so important that when using our Strength and Burly Ultimate Sandbags™ that all bilateral pressing occurs from the top parallel handles. The end flaps are meant to be rolled into the ends of the Ultimate Sandbag and offer the ability to perform some thick grip type of training on exercises such as cleans and rows. Being aware of the structural difference of the Ultimate Sandbag™ over other training implements is important in making sure that you have a long and healthy training experience!

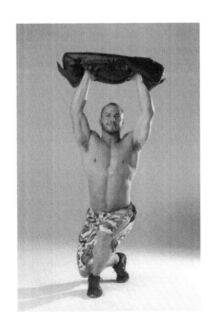

Q: Can I use the Ultimate Sandbag™ mixed in with my other favorite fitness tools?

A: Absolutely! While we believe the DVRT™ program is a phenomenal stand alone system, we also realize that people enjoy using a host of fitness tools and the Ultimate Sandbag™ can blend right in!

However, having said that is important to make sure that you are not making the Ultimate Sandbag™ into something it is not! People often wonder if they can use the Ultimate Sandbag™ to replicate their favorite exercises. Here are some common ones...

Can I swing the Ultimate Sandbag™ like a kettlebell?

No! The Ultimate Sandbag™ does not work well for swings for two reasons. First, the Ultimate Sandbag™ even at more rigid loading levels does not have the same trajectory or motion of a kettlebell being swung. The downward motion in relationship to the handles make for an awkward downward movement. Additionally, the Ultimate Sandbag™ has a completely different dimension making the user to have to compromise their technique in order to perform a swing. The Ultimate Sandbag™ is fantastic for similar movements such as Rotational Lunges and Shoveling.

Can I back squat the Ultimate Sandbag™ like a barbell?

This has actually and yes and no answer to it. It really depends on the weight of the Ultimate Sandbag™ you are using. Lighter USBs can be used to back squat, but are generally part of a complex where back squatting is only part of the exercise. You will never squat as well with the Ultimate Sandbag™ on the upper back as you will in front of the body and the front positions will always challenge the core to a higher degree. The upper back position is sometimes used in exercises such as lunges and step-ups as a counter balance to place people in better lifting postures.

The no answer comes specifically if we are talking about larger weights. Two important reasons for NOT performing heavy back squats with the Ultimate Sandbag™! The first has to be that getting the Ultimate Sandbag™ into such a position would be a high risk proposition for the shoulders and low back considering there is no such thing as a Sandbag Power Rack. That is why for many years old-time strongmen performed Zercher lifts as no barbell power racks existed.

The second reason is that while holding the barbell on the upper back, the trapezius muscles create a "shelf" for the barbell to sit upon. With the Ultimate Sandbag™ in the same position the body cannot create such a shelf and all the load has to be taken by the shoulder and/or the low back. In other words the risk to reward just isn't there! The best reason of all may be the simple fact that by placing the Ultimate Sandbag™ in the front loading positions we work the core harder on every single repetition!

Q: Coach Henkin, I love challenge workouts like those of the 300 model. Do you have anything like that?

A: Yes, we have some fun workouts you can use as a challenge and others that are great programs. While there is a big difference between the two they can still be equally enjoyable, but used for different circumstances.

Fast N' Furious 100

A short and powerful workout that can kick start your conditioning and strength in no time! Follow this ladder of 3/5/7/9 that will give you 25 total repetitions of four different movements. All in all, 100 reps that will definitely challenge your entire fitness!

Exercise	Ladder Series
Rotational Lunge Clean	3/5/7/9
Staggered Clean and Press	3/5/7/9
Zercher Single Leg Deadlift to Balance	3/5/7/9
Two Point Pronated Rows	3/5/7/9

Immortal Workout 1

(Please Check Our Blog at http://UltimateSandbagTraining.com for the Remaining Workouts)

Exercise	Sets	Repetitions
A1. Rotational Lunge Snatch to Forward Lunge	3-5	5/4/3/2/1
A2. Lateral USB™ Drag to T Push-up	3-5	2/4/6/8/10
B1. Zercher Goodmorning to Zercher Squat	3-4	40 Seconds of Work 20 Seconds of Rest

Exercise	Sets	Repetitions
B2. Golf Swing	3-4	40 Seconds of Work 20 Seconds of Rest
B3. Arm Extended Overhead Scissor Side Planks	3-4	40 Seconds of Work 20 Seconds of Rest

Q: What do the letters and numbers mean in all your workouts?

A: Exercises of the same letters mean that they are performed in a circuit manner or supersetted. The numbers simply mean the order in which they are performed. Make sure that you complete all the sets of the circuit or superset series of the workout before moving onto other aspects. Equally important make sure to try not to alter the order of exercises as this will impact the outcome of the workout.

An Ultimate Sandbag™ Success Story

Nine years was the time I spent living in constant pain. It was 2008, I met Josh Henkin and was introduced to a style of training I had never known or saw before. I had always considered myself an athlete. I trained to be apart of the Olympic swimming team until shoulder injuries set me back and would not allow it. I knew what training was about, I knew about the two a days, the six day a week training sessions, I knew what it took to be at the top.

It was my athletic background, that lead me to pursue a degree in physical therapy. It was in my first year of graduate school when I was stretching a patient and I felt my back just give out, the pain was so intense it felt like lightening running down my leg, I had never felt pain like this in my life.

I received an MRI and was told I had the spine of an eighty year old women, about five disc herniations, arthritis and nerve root impingement. The doctors chalked it up to poor genetics and the intense training I had through the years. Not the greatest news for a 21year old.

So I took it upon myself to start my "therapy". I was going to be a therapist, I could do this! I did my stretches, my pelvic tilts and every core exercise in the book. I did everything I was taught in order to "fix" low back pain. Over the course of the next year, the intense pain eventually went away, but the constant dull ache in my low back and legs remained no matter what I did. I continued training the way I knew how, treating my back with conventional physiotherapy methods. Nothing helped. I thought I would just have to live with pain until it got to the point I had to do something more invasive.

I was wrong…I met Josh. At this point I had been a physical therapist for about five years and had continued to find ways to relieve my pain. I started training with Josh, training a way I never had seen before. I had never trained in the manner Josh talked to me about. I didn't know what to think at first, I was so used to walking into a gym and doing "legs" one day, "arms" the next and my hour of cardio. How was I to benefit from this training? How was anyone to benefit from this training?

I found out really quickly how. I could not move, I couldn't even perform a body weight squat without pain shooting down my legs; it was frustrating not to be able to perform the movements. It was frustrating to be in constant pain. Josh introduced the

Ultimate Sandbag™ to me as a way to "teach" my body to move again. It took some time, it didn't happen over night, but it happened!

Some might ask how could Ultimate Sandbag™ Training fix your low back problems? I had tried everything up until now but I never retaught my body to move. Movements like the bear hug squat allowed me to become more upright with my posture and allowed me to load my body in a way that didn't aggravate my symptoms. I used to squat with a bar on my back and the compression was too great and would send pain right down my legs. It allowed me to load my body in a way that was pain free. I had never worked with a dynamic implement before and felt muscles turn on that I never felt before. I felt myself getting stronger than I ever had been.

Fast-forward to the present day (three years later)… I can move without out pain, I can train hard without pain, and I can honestly say it was two things that got me here. Josh Henkin and his DVRT™ system and the Ultimate Sandbag™. His system has taught me to move again and move pain free, something that I had tried to do for so many years.

I could not be more proud of what Josh has accomplished, this book compiles many years of hard work, dedication and innovation. I know Josh has put his heart and soul into creating this system, and I can honestly say it works!

- Jessica Bento, MS, P.T.

For More On Sandbag Training visit:

ULTIMATESANDBAGTRAINING.COM

Join Us On Facebook
At facebook.com/ultimatesandbagtraining

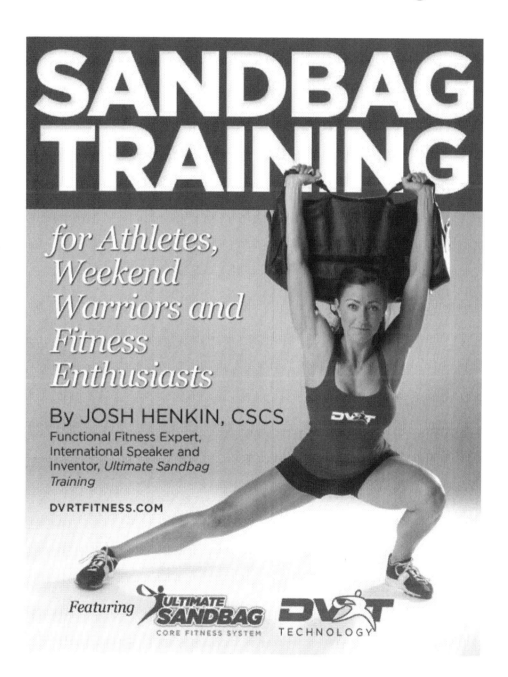

Made in the USA
Lexington, KY
07 August 2012